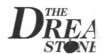

Designed by:
Calm Collective
Churchill Heath Farm
Kingham
Chipping Norton
OX7 6UJ

Published by:
TDS Spirit

Printed by:
Lightening Source UK Ltd.

ISBN: 978-1-9999543-0-7

THE DREAM STONE

A fictional tale about Sam, the Dream Stone and his best friend, Meriel from Oxfordshire. Inspired by real events during Meriel's Dream Stone Triathlon and her other valued personal experiences while living with the Nemaline Myopathy condition. Meriel and her team organised and accomplished their Dream Stone Triathlon Challenge in August 2016. Team MAP Nemaline took Meriel's Dream Stone (Sam) to Snowdon Summit, passing the Dream Stone over water, road and track. Dreams and goals have been accomplished by all, raising an overwhelming amount for charity in only three months.

Written by Meriel and her carer, Anna-Marie. Illustrated by Meriel and her elder brother Miles. Including photographs taken by Team MAP Nemaline.

ACKNOWLEDGEMENTS

Meriel would like to thank her triathlon team, collectively known as Team MAP Nemaline. Their continued encouragement and inspiration has taken Meriel's enthusiasm and positivity to another level. She often refers to her triathlon experiences in her school work which has boosted her self-belief.

Team MAP Nemaline is a growing team of people that support Meriel throughout her life. Family, medical teams, academic staff including pastoral support, and not forgetting the sporting heroes who inspire her. Meriel would like to thank you for simply being her friend, it means a lot to her. She wouldn't be where she is today without you all. Thank you.

A special thank you to everyone who had faith and supported them throughout the writing of this story.

All royalties for MAP Nemaline and for more information visit:

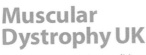
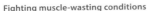

Muscular Dystrophy UK
Fighting muscle-wasting conditions

MAP Nemaline
www.musculardystrophyuk.org/map-nemaline

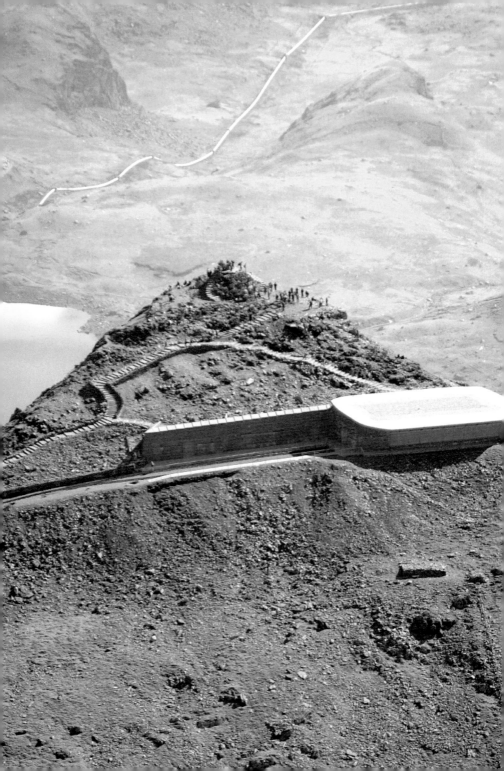

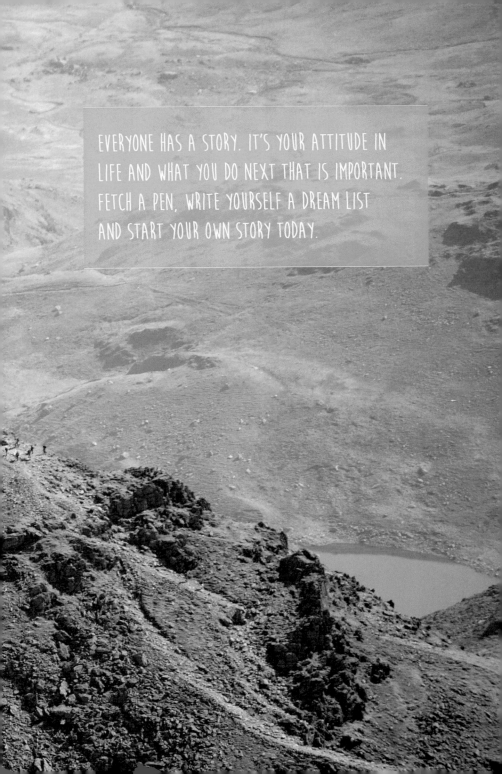

EVERYONE HAS A STORY. IT'S YOUR ATTITUDE IN
LIFE AND WHAT YOU DO NEXT THAT IS IMPORTANT.
FETCH A PEN, WRITE YOURSELF A DREAM LIST
AND START YOUR OWN STORY TODAY.

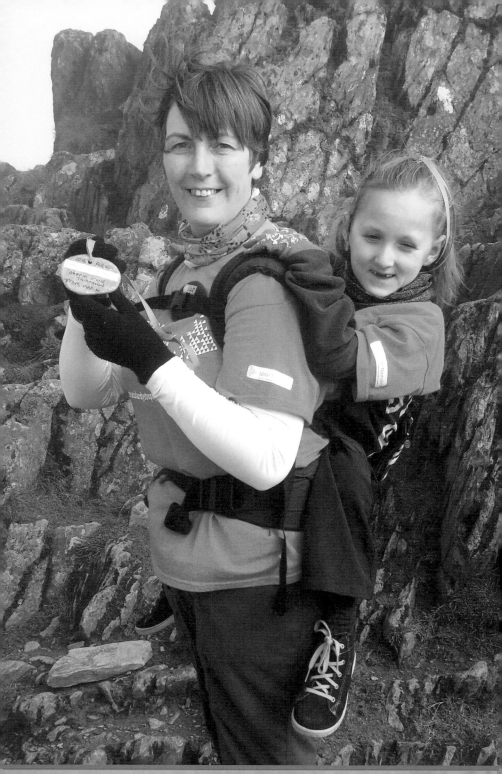

CONTENTS

Muscular Dystrophy UK
Fighting muscle-wasting conditions

MAP Nemaline
www.musculardystrophyuk.org/map-nemaline

CHAPTER 1
DREAM LISTS AND FRIENDS

"I can't see anything, it's too foggy!" squealed Meriel over the noise of the icy wind. The wind and dense fog nipped at her face and made her eyes water. Poppins was also suffering; her legs were weak with fear that she may trip on the steep cobbled steps and tumble down the mountain side with Meriel on her back.

Who would have thought that only three months before, this challenge was just a crazy idea shared between a teacher, a seven-year-old girl, her carer and a stone?

It all began with a stone that wanted a new home. His name was Sam. He lived in a pretty little fishing village in Cornwall, near the highest rock on the beach. He wasn't very happy. Sam had lived on that part of the beach for years. For many summers, he watched children at Sailor Club whilst their parents enjoyed being out on the wild sea. He longed for some adventure and a new home. But how? Sam was a stone with no legs. He depended on someone moving him. "Hey Sam, why are you crying? What's wrong?" squawked his seagull friend.

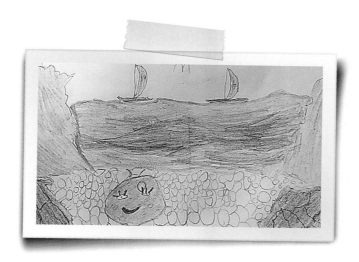

"Oh Gavin, I am so fed up with this beach. The smell of fish is horrible, it's too noisy, the waves crashing on the rocks keep me awake at night; I am extremely tired, I just want some peace and quiet." Sam explained to Gavin that he wanted to be somewhere where he could see the whole world. He wanted to feel the whispering wind, breathe the fresh air, see the rolling hills, the sea and everything in between. Peace and quiet.

Gavin had an idea "Sam, why don't I take you to find a new home? I could carry you in my beak and we could fly."

Sam was delighted "What? Would you really take me to a mountain top so that I can see the world? The fresh mountain air? Flying up in the air like a bird?" He was very excited and wriggled into position, which allowed Gavin to pick him up with his beak.

Gavin and Sam set off on their adventure. They had an amazing time, they flew up above the harbour and around Gavin's nest on the lighthouse roof. They swooped down to see seals bathing on the rocks. Sam was thrilled; he had never seen such wonderful sights. Gavin had seen some boats in the distance, he flapped his wings slightly faster and the wind carried them both out to sea.

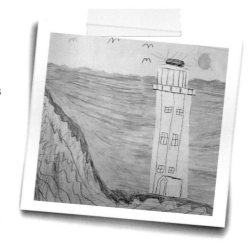

Sam was so excited that he jiggled up and down. He shouted to Gavin and asked him what was happening, but as Gavin tried to answer, Sam slipped to the very front of his beak "...arghhhhh!" cried Sam. "Help me, I can't swim, please don't drop me."

Gavin had tried his best to wriggle him back into a safe position but the wind got stronger and a gust of wind blew Gavin so hard that he lost control. Gavin struggled to keep his beak clamped around Sam, he became so dizzy when he spun around and around that he crashed into a boat sail and lost his grip. Sam had fallen and had slid down the sail, he yelled "Hheeeeellppp!" but Gavin had gone head first through the windblown sail. He kicked his webbed orange feet and had desperately wriggled to try and break free. Sliding down the sail had broken his fall and luckily Sam hadn't landed in the sea, he had fallen into a bag that belonged to a couple who were out sailing for the day.

On returning to shore, the couple went to collect their children from Sailor Club. The children had been collecting beautiful shells and interesting stones.

"Let's go children, time for dinner and we still need to pack our things into the car. It's a long drive home to Oxfordshire," called their father as he stumbled over the shingles.

"Oh Dad" groaned the children, who had really enjoyed collecting their treasures. Meriel had collected lots of shells of different shapes and sizes. She refused to throw any away and asked to put them in his bag so she could take them all home.

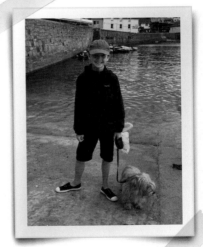

When they got back to their accommodation, their father packed their bags whilst Miles walked the dog. "Can I please take my shells out of the bag?" asked Meriel. She wanted to choose her favourite shell to hold during the journey back to Oxfordshire. When Meriel pulled out her father's belongings she found all the shells on the bottom of the bag. Sam was scared, he had to keep very quiet when Meriel's little hand reached forward and picked him up. "Look at this cool stone" smiled Meriel. "It's very smooth and look, it has a hole, I could make it into a necklace." Meriel spent a long time dusting away the sand to make all the shells nice and clean.

Meriel was delighted to have found a new stone and she kept it in her pocket during dinner. Every so often she put her hand in her pocket and stroked Sam. Sam was worried, not because he was scared of Meriel, but he couldn't help but wonder what had happened to his friend Gavin. When Sam had fallen into the bag he didn't see that Gavin had managed to escape the windy sail and had flown back to his nest on the lighthouse to recover from his frightening ordeal. Thankfully Meriel's caring hands had made Sam feel safe. She seemed like a nice gentle girl who wouldn't have hurt a fly. He felt so relieved after such an adventurous day.

After dinner, they set off on the long journey home, Meriel clutching her new favourite stone.

It was very late and dark when they arrived back home at Oxford. Meriel's mother carried a sleepy girl up to bed and knowing how much she adored her new stone, tucked Sam under the covers.

"Psst, psst, are you awake?"

"Mmmmm?" yawned Meriel, when she heard a whispering voice as she woke up in the morning.

"My name is Sam, thank you so much for bringing me with you."

Meriel thought it was a dream, her stone spoke to her! "Sam?" she yawned.

"Yes, I am Sam, I lived on the beach in Cornwall" explained Sam. He continued to tell her about what had happened and how his brave friend Gavin had tried to take him to find a new home up on a mountain.

Sam felt so sad telling Meriel his story that he actually had a little cry. "Now I will never get to the top of the mountain. Please could I stay here with you?" Meriel took Sam in her small hand and gave him a cuddle. Everyone feels better after one of Meriel's magic cuddles.

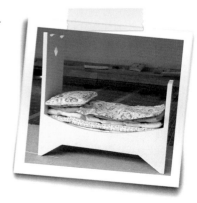

Meriel searched in her toy box to find Sam a little bed that she thought he would like. After a long time thinking where to put the bed, Meriel and Sam decided to keep it over by the swimming pool. This way he would feel like he was at the beach, but without the noisy waves. It was cosy and warm, and thankfully did not smell of fish.

Sam was delighted with his new home. He enjoyed living at the pool and he also encouraged Meriel with her swimming.

Several weeks passed and Sam was very happy, they became great friends. As time passed though, as much as Sam loved Meriel and his new life in Oxfordshire, he still felt a longing in his heart to be upon a mountain so he could see the whole world.

One afternoon Meriel noticed Sam wasn't his normal cheery self. "Sam, you look sad, shall we decorate you? It might cheer you up?" suggested Meriel who always had great ideas. Sam asked to be painted orange like the Cornish sunset, just like the one he used to watch every night back home. Meriel tried to make Sam feel better by telling him about her Dream List.

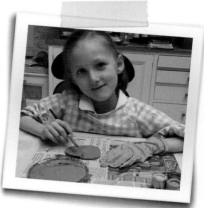

"What's a Dream List?" asked Sam.

"Well, my friend Anna-Marie helps me to think of things that I want to do or try in my lifetime. When I have tried it, I tick it off my list and take lots of photographs for memories. Anyone can have a Dream List, even you! It's such a good feeling when you achieve your dream." Meriel shared a few things on her list with Sam. "I really want to meet an Olympian and touch a polar bear." Meriel encouraged Sam to think of things for his list. After several seconds of thoughtful silence, they both wished out loud. "Go up a mountain." Their eyes met with great excitement when they realised that they both wanted to do the same thing.

"Whenever Anna-Marie walks up a hill or mountain, she always takes a stone. It's a tradition to put a stone in your pocket, take it all the way to the top and then you place it on a cairn", explained Meriel.

You can be my stone Sam, let's do it!" said Meriel with her 'have a bash' attitude. "But how?" questioned Sam "We can't walk!"

Meriel was quick to respond "Maybe I can't walk by myself, but I have Anna-Marie, she tries to help me make my dreams come true" smiled Meriel confidently. "My friends and I call her 'Poppins', after Mary Poppins the magical Nanny."

Meriel and Sam had more in common than they realised as walking is very hard for Meriel, she has a weak muscle condition and struggles to walk. "It's called 'Nemaline Myopathy' Sam, no one really knows what that is because it is so rare, so I just tell people that I have weak muscles." Meriel suggested to Sam that they go up a mountain together.

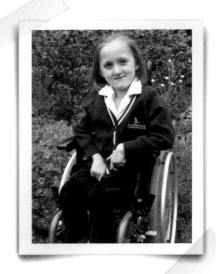

"Sam, my 'Little Dream Stone' we can really do this, if you want to?"

"I will be sad to leave you, but I really think I need to add the mountain to my Dream List, it may be the only quiet place where I can see the whole world." Meriel set to it and asked Poppins to help them.

"Don't worry Meriel, I will make it my mission to get you to the top of a mountain," Poppins said reassuringly.

Poppins had several ideas even though Meriel found it difficult to walk. She could use a ski lift or a cable car in Scotland, but they eventually decided to go up Snowdon by train because it is the highest mountain in England and Wales, 1,085 metres high. Meriel also finds travelling long distances uncomfortable, so they decided to enjoy the Welsh experience nearer home.

One day, Meriel told a teacher at her school about their challenge to take her Little Dream Stone friend up a mountain. Mr Kruze thought it was a fantastic idea and asked to join them on their adventure.

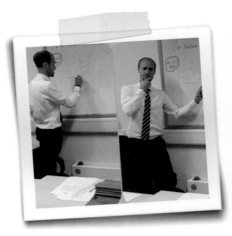

Poppins and Mr Kruze both believe that goals and challenges are important for everyone to become the best that they can be.

Unbeknown to Poppins, when she planned the trip, Mr Kruze's brain was whizzing with ideas to make the trip extra special. One morning Mr Kruze approached Meriel and asked: "How would you like to be part of the best duathlon team ever?" Mr Kruze continued to explain what a duathlon was. His idea involved him cycling 174 miles with a friend from the school all the way to Snowdon in Wales, before heading up the mountain. "Mr Kruze, you are crazy, Crazy-Kruze," exclaimed Poppins to his crazy idea.

Sam was concerned: "Oh my, how will you manage that?" Mr Kruze however, was a bit of a fitness fan and super fit. They often saw him running from task to task at school. "That explains why you are the same shape as a runner bean," joked Sam.

Mr Kruze knew it was a tough, but realistic goal to cycle from Kitebrook to Llanberis, the town at the base of Snowdon. Meriel agreed to do the second part of the duathlon and take Sam up the mountain. Poppins would piggy back them to the very top to touch the trig point. Sam was extremely excited, "I am going to my dream home" he exclaimed.

"Hang on, why don't we turn it into three challenges? Is that called a triathlon?" suggested Meriel. "I could swim, couldn't I? I have been practicing." Sam was impressed that Meriel wanted to make the challenge even harder.

"You may not be as strong as a Welsh Dragon Meriel, but you certainly have the heart of one," smiled Poppins proudly.

From then on, they were collectively known as 'Team MAP Nemaline'. Team MAP-N. The name was inspired from their chosen charity, MAP Nemaline, and it had to include everyone and all the events. When Mr Kruze and Meriel trained, lots had been happening behind the scenes. Promotional posters and t-shirts were designed. Social media pages and a donation site were all set up to allow friends to follow their adventure. It was a very exciting time.

Sam believed that it was a great charity to support because Meriel's parents had created the Family Fund with help from Muscular Dystrophy UK. All the money raised helps scientists find out more about Meriel's weak muscle condition, Nemaline Myopathy. Within the first weekend of fundraising over a £1,000 was raised.

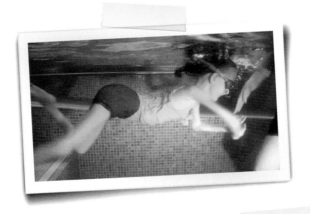

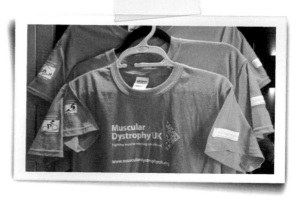

CHAPTER 2
READY, STEADY, TRAINING

One afternoon as Meriel practiced in the pool, she and Poppins discussed what swim challenge she would do for the triathlon. "A challenge is something that you can't do yet, an activity that is a bit tricky to achieve, but not impossible with hard work," explained Poppins. "The harder you work, the more amazing you will feel when you achieve your goal." Poppins suggested a few swimming activities using floats, such as swimming two lengths of the pool.

"Two lengths? No way, I will drown. I know, why don't I swim one length with no floats in the deep side?"

They decided to try and swim the length that day, then they could find out how much training she needed to do, or if indeed it was far too difficult. That's just what they did.

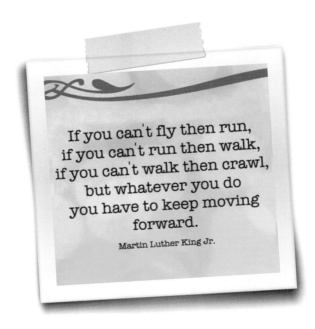

If you can't fly then run,
if you can't run then walk,
if you can't walk then crawl,
but whatever you do
you have to keep moving
forward.

Martin Luther King Jr.

JUST A SIMPLE BREATH

Meriel's condition makes lung activity hard because of the weak surrounding muscles. Simple things like singing and shouting were tough when she was younger. Particularly as she only has one and a half lung capacity and gets out of breath very easily. Meriel uses a Ventilator Nippy machine to assist with her breathing during the night or if she is ill during the day and a Cough Assist machine when she has a simple cold to assist clearing the phlegm and to boost her lungs by inflating them. When out and about she uses a lightweight portable device that also inflates her lungs (LVR bag).

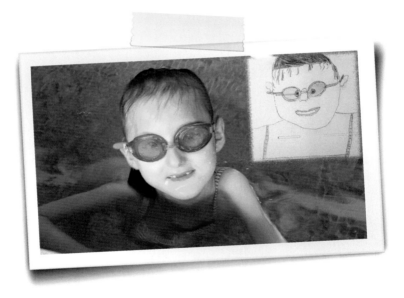

"PUFFS" struggled Meriel after three strokes as Poppins scooped her out of the water.

"There you go," Poppins said when she administered some rescue puffs of air from her hospital gadget. Several puffs later, Meriel felt relaxed and ready to go again.

"You're doing great," said Sam with an envious tone, he couldn't quite believe how brave she was. He wished that he could swim but he would sink straight to the bottom.

Meriel swam underwater when she didn't use her floats. She needed help to come to the surface to breathe. Due to her very slim and weak build she couldn't float unaided. Poppins scooped her out of the water to recover. Sam was on stopwatch duty, he timed Meriel's first attempt to swim the length of the pool (ten metres), "Twenty minutes!" shouted Sam to the far end of the pool.

"Oh, I will never do it," sighed Meriel. Poppins reassured her.

"Meriel, it may take you one hour to swim your length, it doesn't matter as long as you try your best, the challenge isn't to do it quickly." Meriel understood and kept practicing.

During the summer holidays Meriel went swimming a lot with her family. "Wow, Meriel you are getting so good," said Sam excitedly. He was dreaming of the hills and mountains every night now. In one of his dreams an eagle flew high above his new home and screeched which reminded him of his seagull friend Gavin. Things do happen for a reason, thought Sam. "If Gavin hadn't dropped me I wouldn't be here with you preparing for the triathlon."

Meriel agreed with Sam, "Yes you are right, if I didn't have weak muscles, I wouldn't have met Prince Harry last year," she said with a big smile. "I think he would be proud knowing that I was taking on this triathlon challenge."

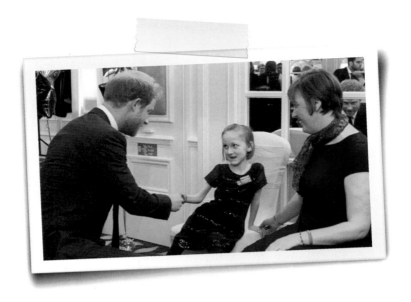

WELLCHILD AWARDS 2015

Meriel was nominated by her teacher, Mrs Ella, for WellChild's Inspirational Child Award in 2015, which she won. His Royal Highness Prince Harry is the Patron of the WellChild charity.

He presented the award to her on stage. Prince Harry and Meriel spoke before the ceremony, they discussed her love for swimming and football. The whole experience was the first major boost of confidence that Meriel had had, a life changing moment and an experience that no one will ever forget.

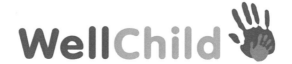

Team MAP-N trained hard over the summer months. Poppins planned the trip and researched various piggyback slings to use with Meriel to ensure that she was comfortable. They eventually borrowed one from The Oxford Sling Library.

If Mr Kruze was not on his bicycle he was in the gym. He bought a new red helmet, that pleased Meriel as both Mr Kruze and Meriel are keen Arsenal football fans and red is their team colour.

One glorious day Mr Kruze had been oiling his bicycle chain and fitting new brakes, he checked that his bicycle was in tip-top condition. Before he had a chance to tighten up the last few bolts on his brakes, his friend Ross called him on the telephone. "Is it that time already?" shouted Mr Kruze, he had lost track of the time and forgotten that he had a very special date to attend. He dropped everything and rushed upstairs to get himself spruced up. She must have been a special lady because he even pinned a flower to his best jacket. Once ready, he jumped over his tools and with the biggest smile jumped into his car and zoomed off.

Meanwhile in the pool, Sam and Meriel's big brother, Miles had been of great support. Meriel's breaststrokes and 'froggy legs' had improved but most importantly, she wasn't scared of swimming in the deep side any more. When on holiday in Scotland she tried other kinds of training like cycling and she even tried bagpipes. "This is good for my lungs," she joked with Sam. Poor Sam listened to the painful squawk of the bagpipes. "Oh dear" he moaned as he pulled a weird face, "that sounds awful."

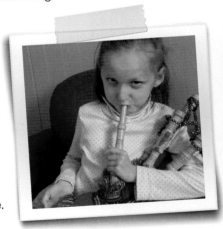

As the challenge date grew closer Meriel and Sam started to worry. "Poppins, what if I become ill? What if I get a cold?" she asked with a sad face.

"Don't worry Meriel, we shall carry on with 'The Magic 5' and keep strong. Hopefully the bugs will be too scared to attack," reassured Poppins. But the truth is, bugs were out of Poppins control.

THE MAGIC 5

Getting a simple cold can be very serious, if Meriel gets a very bad cold it can lead to time in hospital. When Poppins started to care for Meriel she introduced "The Magic 5". The five things that everyone, even Olympians should do every day to encourage them to stay healthy. Fresh air: food and water: exercise: sleep and the most important - lots of giggles. This was the first motivational tool that Anna-Marie initiated every day.

"In case you are too poorly to travel, I will make you a deal," smiled Poppins.

Poppins promised Meriel and Sam that if Meriel was too poorly to travel to Wales, she would rise to the challenge and walk up the whole of Snowdon herself with Sam hanging around her neck all the way to the summit. "All it takes is faith, trust and a little bit of pixie dust!" smiled Poppins, recalling a good luck card that was sent to Meriel. However, everyone hoped and prayed that Meriel would stay healthy and manage to do the challenge with the team.

Poppins thought that she had better start training herself. Dream Lists motivate you to do things that you may not have tried. Preparing for her family summer holiday in Scotland, Poppins packed her walking boots and outdoor gear, she walked several hills during her holiday.

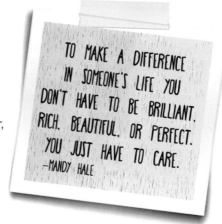

TO MAKE A DIFFERENCE IN SOMEONE'S LIFE YOU DON'T HAVE TO BE BRILLIANT. RICH. BEAUTIFUL. OR PERFECT. YOU JUST HAVE TO CARE.
—MANDY HALE

CHAPTER 3
SINK OR SWIM?

It was a beautiful hot and sunny day in Oxfordshire, the most perfect day for the Dream Stone Triathlon. Meriel started with her ten metre swim challenge.

"Meriel, Meriel, come on it's time to get up and get ready for your guests," encouraged her mother, who was up very early and had already baked a cake for the guests.

They had invited a few neighbours to watch, offering Meriel moral support and to stay for cake afterwards as a way to say thank you.

Sam and the family knew how nervous Meriel was. Poppins knew how hard she had trained and was very proud of her attitude. "I said I was going to do it, so I am!" was Meriel's response when Poppins had suggested an easier challenge. She was a very determined and strong spirited young girl who always tried her best.

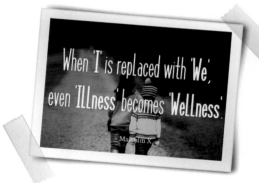

When 'I' is replaced with 'We', even 'Illness' becomes 'Wellness'.

© Malcolm X

When the guests arrived Meriel however, had shrunk from a confident swimming penguin to a shy little goldfish. "I'm scared," she whispered to Poppins. Poppins knew from experience that it was scary attempting a new challenge, especially doing it in front of others, but she also knew how Meriel would feel when she completed her goal with family and friends around her.

Sam tried to make Meriel relax and joked about how he was going to jump in the pool and splash Mr Kruze. However, Sam had actually fallen in, when he was being silly. Miles swam quickly to his rescue, scooped him up and held Sam high above his head when he came out of the water as if Sam was a gold medal. "Ewww! Why are you all slimy?" shrieked Miles "yuk!"

Poppins and Meriel had tears of laughter because of the expression on his face. "Oh, Miles you are hilarious, you don't like sticky fingers, do you?" Poppins laughed so much that her tummy muscles ached and tears trickled down her cheek.

Miles was repulsed by the strange goo on his fingers. "Take him, take him," he pleaded as he handed sticky Sam to Poppins.

"Is he dead?" Meriel asked with great concern.

"I am meeeeelllltttting" mumbled Sam, who didn't like the strange sticky feeling either.

"He's okay Meriel." Poppins had tried to control her giggles and take things more seriously when Miles tried to wipe the slime from his hands.

Unfortunately, the warm water had melted the protective glaze over Sam's beautiful sunset colour. "But we even tested it Poppins, I don't understand."

"We only tested it for cool mountain rain Meriel," explained Poppins.

"Disgusting…," said Miles with an emerging grin.

When Mr Kruze and his new wife Jennie heard of the sticky drama they joined in the laughter and it actually helped everyone relax, they were all slightly nervous, thinking: "Would Meriel sink or swim?".

The pool area had been decorated with flags, balloons and a good luck banner made by one of the guests. Meriel's favourite songs from the WellChild Awards were in the CD player ready for her to swim to. Sam was stationed at the end of the pool with the stopwatch and Miles was ready to video the special event.

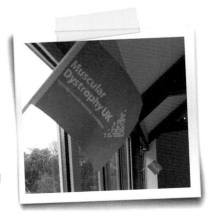

The nervous silence was deafening, it even made Poppins nervous, she told everyone to "Talk amongst yourselves," before she gave Meriel a last boost of confidence.

"Why do I keep smiling?" Meriel whispered: "I can't stop"

Poppins smiled and explained that it was only her nerves that made her smile and there was nothing to fear. "Try and enjoy it Meriel, you can only do your best."

"Are you ready? Let's do this," smiled Poppins and the music started.

Poppins gave Meriel an encouraging secret wink just as the song had started. The first few beats of Jess Glynne's song 'Hold my Hand' gave everyone goosebumps, it always made Meriel and Poppins' hearts flutter because it reminded them of the WellChild awards. She had chosen the perfect song.

Off she kicked. Meriel's first four strokes were fantastic, far better than during training. Poppins and Meriel had constant eye contact throughout the swim. Poppins scooped Meriel up to allow her to breathe safely.

Suddenly out of the nervous silence she heard a familiar voice: "Great start Meriel, good start." It was Mr Kruze. Meriel smiled when she heard him, but then she struggled to stop smiling and had forgotten to close her mouth when she started her second set of strokes. Luckily Poppins' super quick reactions pulled her out of the water in a split second. Meriel and Poppins laughed, she was reminded to keep her mouth closed and off she swam again.

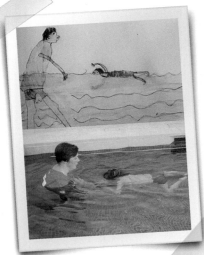

They couldn't believe how little recovery time Meriel needed after breaths. Meriel had kicked her hardest that day. When she reached halfway,

Poppins screeched, "I'm getting excited!" Sam was also watching in disbelief, Meriel had taken twenty minutes when she first attempted to swim the length. That day it looked like she may have achieved a new personal best!

Her spectators got excited as well, they shouted encouragement from the side lines.

Knowing how tired she had become, Poppins growled: "Come on, let's go, push it!" which helped Meriel to dig deeper. Poppins already had tear-filled eyes with pride, so when Meriel completed her length and was scooped up to the pool side to recover, Poppins struggled to hold back her tears, she focused on helping Meriel put on her orange Team MAP Nemaline t-shirt.

It was like being at the WellChild awards ceremony all over again, many photos and poses, everyone was very proud and fought back their tears as Mr Kruze presented Meriel with a certificate of achievement. Most importantly Meriel was proud of herself, even though she was exhausted, she continued to smile. Sam glanced at the stopwatch: "Mmmm this can't be right," he thought.

"Meriel you will never guess your time," shouted Sam, "I just can't believe it!" It went silent and everyone waited in suspense "Four minutes, YES, four minutes, you have totally smashed your record Meriel." Everyone was delighted. Meriel was just glad it was over, she was very happy but also exhausted.

After they celebrated in the sunshine and discussed the next stage of the Dream Stone Triathlon, Sam had to say goodbye to Meriel's family.

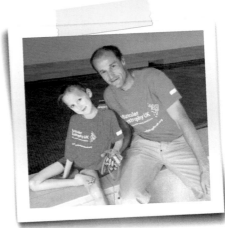

He was very sad yet excited when he embarked on the next stage of the triathlon with Mr Kruze. Sam's ribbon came in handy, as he travelled most of the one hundred and seventy four miles around Mr Kruze's neck like a necklace to keep him safe and warm.

"Don't worry Sam, I will see you soon, Mr Kruze will look after you. I will see you in Wales for our last part of the triathlon together," said Meriel as she gave him a little comforting kiss.

When Mr Kruze left with Sam, Meriel felt like there was a hole in her little heart. She didn't sleep well that night, unsure if it was because of the exciting day completing her swim challenge or because she missed Sam. I need to get used to being without Sam, thought Meriel because soon I will need to say goodbye for real and leave my little Dream Stone at the top of the mountain. She rubbed her tear-filled eyes and snuggled into her bed to sleep.

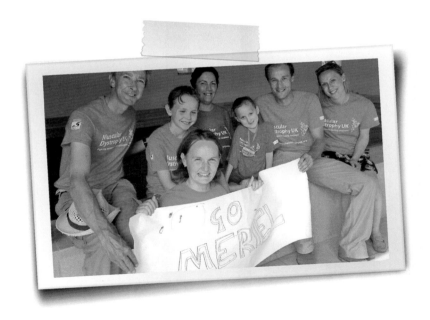

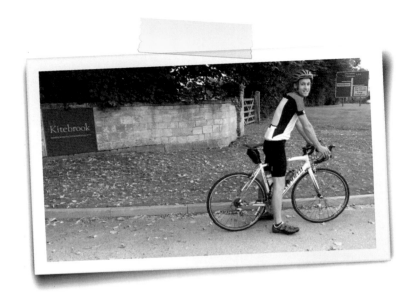

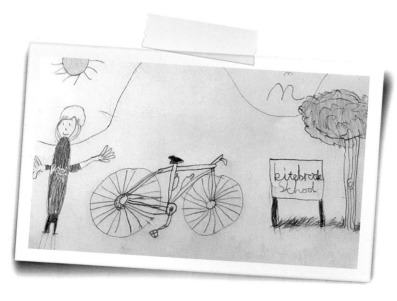

CHAPTER 4
BIONIC BOYS

During the following days Mr Kruze, Jennie and her brother Ross (Mr Kruze's cycle buddy) all made their final preparations. Mr Kruze and Ross had talked a lot about which route to take. The men wanted a scenic and challenging yet safe route.

Jennie had cooked up a storm in the kitchen the night before, she made lots of healthy energy bars for them to eat during their journey. She was also the team's designated 'Safety Driver'. Should there have been any issues, injuries or accidents she would have been nearby to support the team. Jennie's most important job was to find the best cafes for a nice cup of Earl Grey tea and cake, after all, they had to keep their energy levels topped up.

Sam had spent most of the night watching the men sort out their equipment in the garage. The bicycles were their pride and joy; every polish and buff was given with great care and attention as if they were babies.

The morning of the cycle was rather exciting; Jennie had been on the case to ensure that the men hadn't forgotten anything (especially Sam). "Here you are, you can't forget this special little guy," she said as she hung an excited Sam around Mr Kruze's neck like a gold medal.

"You will be safe here Sam. Cosy and very warm and you will have such a great view speeding down the hills with me" said Mr Kruze as he climbed upon his bicycle and tucked Sam into his t-shirt.

Sam was nervous, he had never been on a bicycle before. At least I am not going to melt again like I did in Meriel's pool thought Sam. Remembering that day made him giggle.

"Oi Sam! Stop giggling, you're tickling me and making me wiggle!" chuckled Mr Kruze as he tried to control his wiggly zig-zag steering. They left school very early in the morning to try and miss the busy bank holiday traffic.

Everyone had been rather concerned about Ross, he had strained his knee and it wasn't fully healed. Jennie was on standby in case of an emergency, but the men had a good start and stopped for a stretch and a drink after several miles along the deserted road.

"What kind of animal is that?" asked Sam as he looked towards the field. "Looks like one of those hairy Highland cows that I saw in Scotland with Meriel."

"No Sam, it is a Shetland pony, that little fella actually belongs to my sister," explained Mr Kruze. "Come on Pumpkin," he called. "Come and get your breakfast carrot, I know you're not allowed too many but I packed a couple especially for you."

PUMPKIN

Pumpkin is a rescue pony who was abandoned before his birthday in very poor condition. He was found in a village running away from several dogs and was nearly hit by a car. A charity called Sue Pike Equestrian and Animal Rescue (SPEAR) supported his rehabilitation and nursed him back to good health. Pumpkin continues to live a happy life with Mr Kruze's family where he has learned better manners within the group, but still shows his cheeky, naughty side sometimes.

"He is partial to a game of football Sam; do you want to watch?" laughed Mr Kruze.

Ross and Mr Kruze jumped over the gate, they had fun as they kicked around an old muddy football that they found wedged under the hedge. The pony bucked and neighed with excitement. Pumpkin moved in towards Mr Kruze's foot and nudged the ball confidently with his nose.

"Well, I have never seen anything like it," said Sam amused. "One crazy, miniature football playing pony, Meriel would love him."

Mr Kruze agreed "Yes, he is great fun, but he can be a bit cheeky at times, you need to watch your back or he may take a sneaky nibble."

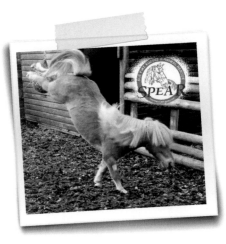

After they had all said goodbye to Pumpkin, they continued on with their journey. Pumpkin continued to call for them. They could still hear him braying like a donkey in the distance as they climbed up another hill.

It had been a glorious day with little traffic and Sam particularly enjoyed the Cotswold scenery. The team made great progress during the first fifty-five miles and even beat Jennie to their lunch rendezvous point. "Hey! You guys must have been going very fast?" Jennie queried with her concerned motherly tone. "You need to take care of your knee Ross." Ross laughed at his 'worry wort sister'.

"Oh, it's okay, that was just a warm up." winked Sam. The men laughed because they knew that they had been naughty, and had pushed their limits, racing each other like boys do.

"Come on 'Bionic Boys', let's go and get a cup of tea," suggested Jennie, laughing at the nickname that she had given the cycle team.

"Yeah a nice comfy seat sounds good," agreed Mr Kruze as he hobbled off his bicycle and waddled like a penguin into the café garden.

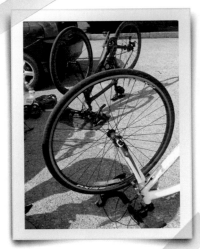

While the team rested, Sam relaxed on the handle bars of Mr Kruze's bicycle and basked like a seal in the warm sunshine. He had been admiring Ross's bicycle, Betsy. She was matt black and looked very expensive.

Sam had seen what great care he took of her; he even put a towel down on the ground when it was placed upside down to get a wheel fixed. The name Betsy doesn't suit this classy, fast machine thought Sam. It reminded him of something; oh yes, Batman, thought Sam. "Ross, your bicycle looks like it belongs to Batman!" chuckled Sam.

"I wonder if it will develop wings when we fly down the hills in Wales," teased Mr Kruze.

Ross, not impressed with their jokes, went over to comfort poor Betsy.

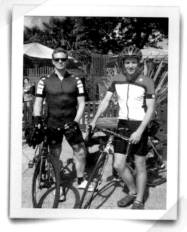

"At least you look after me Betsy, not like this old bone shaker," pointing to Mr Kruze's bicycle. "Who's got the sore bottom now?" retaliated Ross. The team all laughed as they made their preparations for the rest of their journey.

Sam snuggled into Mr Kruze's t-shirt once again and off they cycled.

After several miles of silence, Sam was concerned. "Mr Kruze, are you okay? I can feel your heart and lungs pounding like they are going to burst."

Mr Kruze struggled on the second stretch, the adrenalin from the morning's excitement must have helped him attack those hills, but after lunch he had started to tire.

"Oh Sam, I feel awful, my legs are like heavy rocks and the vibrations from the bumps are going up my arms."

"Shall we stop, then?" suggested Sam.

"No! We've got to keep going, we can't let Meriel down." With this thought Mr Kruze reached for his packet of Strawberry Lace sweets in his pocket, his old faithful friends, to give him the extra boost needed. The smell of his Strawberry Lace sweets had reminded him instantly of the time when he went walking in Tenerife and he only had Strawberry Laces and Digestive biscuits to eat whilst he climbed up a mountain. Not a very sensible idea, thought Sam.

He had kept a steady pace and never gave up. After they had climbed a few more hills, the bionic duo were so relieved when they approached a descending hill at last. "Hold on Sam, this is going to be fun!" cried Mr Kruze.

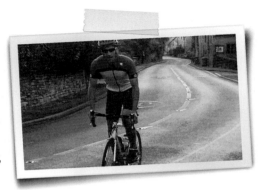

They went faster and faster, the gap between the men extended and the squeals of excitement got louder. When all of a sudden Mr Kruze realized his brakes had unscrewed and dangled dangerously near the spokes of his wheel. Ross had gone too far ahead and didn't hear them shout for help. Now Mr Kruze wished it was his bicycle that had wings, so he had to be brave and tried to make a scary manoeuvre without falling off. "Trust me Sam, I've seen this on the internet, just hold on," he said reassuringly as he tucked Sam back inside his t-shirt.

Mr Kruze reluctantly took his feet off the pedals and as soon as the pedals were free they spun really fast. The 'Bone Shaker' wobbled, Sam was petrified and worried that they may crash. He sobbed quietly to himself. But surprisingly Mr Kruze had regained control and manoeuvred into a faster position. Slowly, he pointed his legs behind and slid his tummy onto the seat and lay flat like Superman's flying position. Luckily, he was still able to steer because there were several potholes as they approached Ross's tail. Sam could tell Mr Kruze was scared because his heart raced and his skin was on fire, like someone had suddenly switched on a heater inside his t-shirt.

"Oh no, not again!" Sam whispered to himself, so not to distract Mr Kruze. "Ewww". Mr Kruze glanced down to his speedometer, he had reached speeds exceeding 44mph, Ross must be going at least 50mph thought Mr Kruze.

Ross, oblivious to the crisis behind him, had continued to sing at the top of his voice. He nearly choked on a random fly that flew into his mouth when Mr Kruze and Sam shot past him.

"Help us!" shouted Mr Kruze.

Ross couldn't quite believe or even understand what he had seen, but his bionic buddy obviously needed some help. So, Ross upped his game and cycled the 'Bat Bike' faster until he caught up. He managed to grab onto Mr Kruze's outstretched foot and slowly applied his brakes and gradually slowed them to a halt.

"Oh, my goodness, that was an awesome ride," grinned Mr Kruze. "Beat you."

Ross couldn't believe it: "What on earth happened?"

When Mr Kruze told Ross about the brakes and his Superman manoeuvre, Sam peeked out of his t-shirt. "Eh, Mr Kruze, there's a problem." There was a confused silence and the men looked puzzled "I've melted, again," Mr Kruze and Ross burst into fits of laughter, which made Sam laugh and relax.

"Don't worry little guy, it's all good," comforted Mr Kruze.

CHAPTER 5
RESCUE AND A MILKSHAKE PLEASE

Mr Kruze wondered how his new brakes could have failed him, then he realised, "Ross! It was my wedding!"

Ross looked confused, "What has the wedding got to do with the bike?"

"Remember? You phoned me because I was late to the church. I was in the middle of attaching my brakes and I never went back to check them," explained Mr Kruze.

Sam interrupted their conversation. "Did you know that not only did you marry Jennie on Meriel's Birthday, but in the same place she had been a bridesmaid the month before?"

"Really? That is a coincidence," agreed Mr Kruze fumbling for his phone.

They phoned Jennie and told her that they had to take a detour via Shrewsbury, to find a bicycle shop to check the bike. Ross asked her to go on an ice hunt for his knee whilst they searched for a bicycle repair shop, as his knee had swollen badly right in front of his eyes. "I think I need to get some ice, quick!" His superhero actions on his Bat Bike must have caused more trauma to his fragile knee. When they got to Shrewsbury they found a very kind mechanic at Stan's Shop, that offered to help them for free and a nearby café gave them some ice. Ross sat with his leg up on a chair to relieve the pain for a while. Mr Kruze didn't complain, he had three milkshakes by the time they left, banana being his favourite.

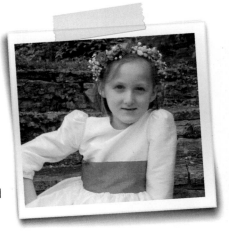

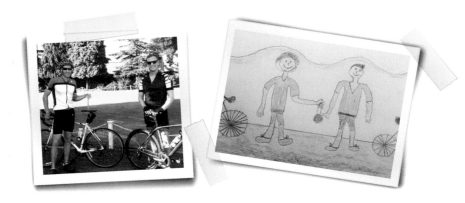

"Surprised he's not fat," commented Sam.

"Apparently, he was when he was a boy," Jennie giggled. "Now he seems to be able to eat anything and everything and he tells me he has two or three puddings most days at school." Jennie chuckled: "I suppose he never stops, he is always on the move."

Sam laughed "Yeah, the Runner Bean."

Once everyone had recovered they returned to their bikes for the last stretch before their accommodation for the night in Oswestry. Both men were relieved that day was almost over. They had covered one hundred and eleven miles since they left the school that morning.

Jennie had invited Sam to travel with her in the car for the last part of the day. He had a great view of the road ahead sitting near the window. They tried to pronounce the road signs when they crossed into Wales. "How people can read them so quickly when driving with English and Welsh directions?" puzzled Sam.

They had arrived at the hotel in Oswestry first. "I feel like I am playing cards with Meriel, which colour will appear first, red or black?" smiled Sam impatiently as they waited, when he suddenly saw a glimmer of red that bobbed up and down. "It's Mr Kruze, with Ross tight on his heels."

Although their legs were numb and bottoms sore, the Bionic Boys felt proud that they had made it this far. The team relaxed and recuperated that night, the hardest day was over.

CHAPTER 6
TEAM MAP-N REUNITE

Back in Oxfordshire Poppins had packed the car with all Meriel's gear. Travelling light is impossible with Meriel due to the various machines that she requires, and then there were the clothes to keep them both warm up the mountain. Poppins packed her own walking gear in case the train up the mountain was cancelled if the weather became too windy. Luckily, they had a Plan B. Poppins would give Meriel a piggyback as far as they could manage. Team MAP Nemaline would place Sam somewhere on the mountain, whether it was at the summit would depend on the weather.

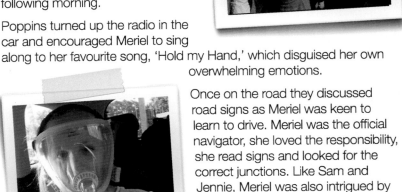

The family had a lump in their throat as they waved Meriel off. It was an emotional morning for them all, who would have ever have thought that Meriel would be at the top of Snowdon the following morning.

Poppins turned up the radio in the car and encouraged Meriel to sing along to her favourite song, 'Hold my Hand,' which disguised her own overwhelming emotions.

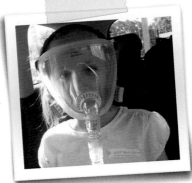

Once on the road they discussed road signs as Meriel was keen to learn to drive. Meriel was the official navigator, she loved the responsibility, she read signs and looked for the correct junctions. Like Sam and Jennie, Meriel was also intrigued by the Welsh sign posts.

Having crossed the border, they played 'Count the Welsh Flags'.
By the time they had reached the hotel they had counted nineteen.

Meriel was adamant that they had to beat the Bionic Boys to the hotel in Llanberis. She kept a look out for Mr Kruze's red Arsenal coloured helmet throughout the whole journey.

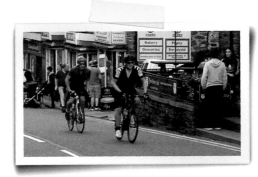

Although the Bionic Boys had climbed steeper hills and struggled along the busy roads with tourists and caravans. They had sixty-five miles left until their destination, but the amazing scenery had kept them motivated.

They stopped for lunch at a delicious farm shop that Jennie had found. The men discussed the remaining route with Sam. "Looks like we have a few nice villages to go through, with a couple of hills, but going up towards the Pen y Pass car park will be the hardest part!" Sam was thrilled when he realised that only three months ago, he had slept on the Cornish beach and listened to the waves every night. He smiled when he imagined being at the top of his Dream Mountain, sleeping under the stars once again. "Ah the whispering wind and fresh air, thanks Team MAP Nemaline," smiled Sam as he thought out loud.

That afternoon with only about ten miles to go, they cycled through a small, yet busy town called Betws y Coed. The men were halfway up a hill where the road had become narrower, the queue of cars had increased by the minute, when there was a sudden loud toot of a car horn. "How dare they toot" shouted Sam. Mr Kruze turned to look only to hear…, "Come on, get those legs moving!" two smiley faces beamed whilst waving out of the car window.

"Meriel" shouted Sam. Poppins pulled over, aware that the men may not stop as they would want to keep up speed to get up the hill. Meriel was excited and had her camera ready. "I knew we would catch them, I knew it!" she said as she clicked her camera, this time of the smiley Bionic Boys who although sweaty and tired, were very pleased to see her.

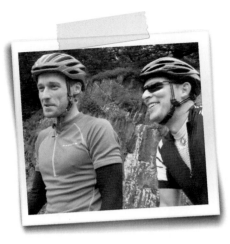

After a quick catch-up and she checked all was okay, Poppins drove off with a toot of her car horn and left the men disappearing in her rear-view mirror.

Further along the road Poppins couldn't help but be concerned for the men when they approached the climb to the Pen y Pass car park. "Oh dear, look at that hill in front Meriel." She drove slowly around the tight, steep corners for fear of the traffic and the sheep that wandered along the road. It would be hard enough to cycle up the hill after such a long journey, but the traffic in the middle of the narrow road filled her heart with fear. When the time came however, the Bionic Boys found their dragon spirit and attacked the climb with gusto, they managed to reach the top safely and stopped to admire the stunning views of the rugged hills, dotted with white specks of sheep in the distance.

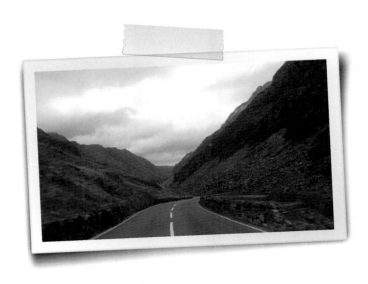

The team loved the journey down the other side. "It's like rally driving," said Meriel. The zig-zag bends were supervised by the rugged mountains that towered above watching over their sheep. The sheep wandered onto the road and didn't seem frightened when cars approached. They would continue to chew their grass until the drivers grew impatient and gave their horn a toot which startled them off the road.

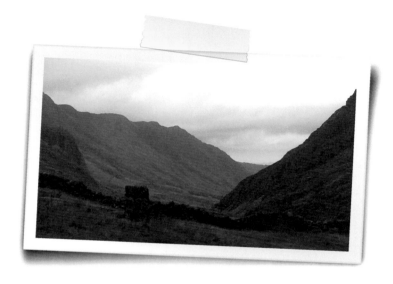

"Wow Poppins, look at the mountains!"

"You have seen nothing yet sweetheart, tomorrow we will see what it looks like from the top." Meriel had enjoyed every part of the journey. She never stopped talking or smiling, apart from when she tried to take a small nap, "I am too excited to sleep." Meriel and Poppins were looking forward to the climb up Snowdon. Poppins was proud of everyone and pleased how everything had come together perfectly. It had been an amazing experience for all of them.

Not long after they arrived at the hotel, they were reunited with their first teammate. "Jennie" squealed Meriel when she spotted her drive into the carpark. All three girls were overjoyed and glad when Team MAP Nemaline were all safely reunited.

MERIEL'S SCOLIOSIS

Completing the Dream Stone Triathalon with the team was something that meant a lot to Poppins and Meriel. Poppins was uncertain if this day would ever happen. Especially at a time of uncertainty regarding which path Meriel's health would take in the future. Her weak muscles and lungs weren't Meriel's only struggle, she developed Scoliosis, which means her spine bends to the side and unfortunately gets worse through time. It has already made it harder to continue with her daily tasks, even standing on her own was becoming no longer possible. An appointment to discuss operating on Meriel's spine was in the diary. Meriel's family were very concerned because of the complications ahead. One year later it was decided that an operation was inadvisable. So, Meriel's spine continues to change and make life more difficult. It affects her eating and breathing, but even with many obstacles in her way Meriel continues to fight, trying her best at school and life in general with a constant twinkle in her eye. When times get tough achieving her goals is so important.

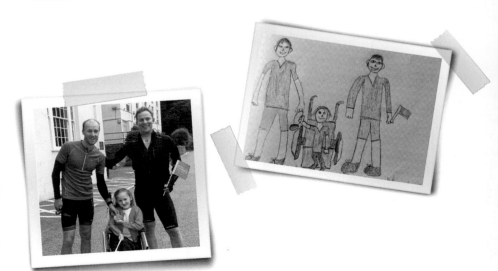

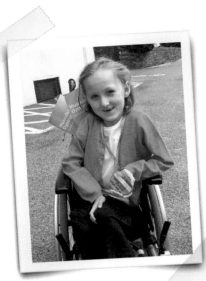

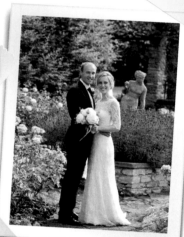

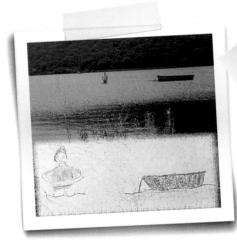

CHAPTER 7
THE UNLUCKY HOURS

When Sam saw Meriel again, he couldn't wait to tell her about their Superman drama and how Jennie had to be nurse again for Ross's knee. "I was terrified Meriel, and guess what happened? I melted, again!" exclaimed Sam.

"Yes, there was goo everywhere," joked Mr Kruze. "Now I understand why Miles was upset, you were all slimy." Everyone laughed.

After returning Sam to Meriel, Mr Kruze brought the bags in from the car. Jennie kept Meriel company showing her wedding photos, she was so pleased to hear that they got married on Meriel's birthday.

Later, the men went for a walk to stretch their painful legs. Ross had a plan, which he hoped would ease his painful knee.

"I am going to paddle in the lake, I think the freezing water will help my sore knee."

"This is going to be hilarious!" chuckled Mr Kruze.

"Can I come?" shouted Sam.

They waddled along until they reached the lakeside. "Okay here goes..," said Ross reluctantly, "Do you want to come in Sam?" Ross held Sam and slowly edged deeper into the lake.

Mr Kruze wasn't so brave and was never very keen on water activities. "I think I'll just stretch out here." Jennie laughed at the pair of the 'Not So Bionic Boys who hobbled about like old men.

"Be careful Ross," pleaded Sam as Ross slipped on the uneven stones deep beneath him. Ross carefully turned around to face his teammates on the shore, when suddenly he felt a tickle behind his knee that made him jump.

"What on earth was that?" he exclaimed, as the tail of a fish brushed his other knee. This time Ross stepped to the side, but he slipped on a boulder and shouted as he heard Sam fall into the lake with a plop. Forgetting his pain Ross grappled under the water and felt around for Sam's ribbon, "Jennie help!" Mr Kruze and Jennie didn't need to think twice, they ran into the lake to where Ross was on all fours desperately hunting for Sam, water splashed everywhere.

After what seemed a long time, Mr Kruze felt Sam's ribbon amongst the rocks and managed to yank him free.

Ross dried Sam carefully on the shore with his towel. "I am really sorry Sam, are you alright?"

"Phew, that was close, but it's all good, at least he didn't melt this time," joked Mr Kruze. The team shook their heads with laughter as they stood dripping wet on the lakeside.

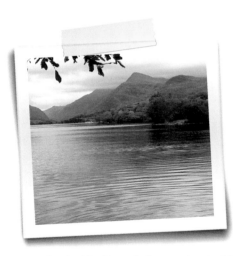

Back at the hotel Meriel glanced out of the window she noticed a group of bedraggled people waddle up the drive. Mr Kruze had his hands in his pockets and scuffed his feet like a naughty schoolboy. "What on earth have you been up to? I thought you were going for a paddle, not a dip?" laughed Poppins as the three very soggy musketeers handed her Sam.

"Don't ask..," sniggered Mr Kruze who hobbled slowly up the stairs wishing the lift hadn't broke down, today of all days. They all went for a nice hot bath and changed out of their soggy rescue clothes.

Hoping to raise spirits Poppins checked the fundraiser website to see how much money they had currently raised for the MAP Nemaline fund. "WOW" she exclaimed, "In two months Meriel we are only twenty pounds short of £14,000." Meriel had no concept of how much that was, but just smiled and popped another chip in her mouth. They were interrupted by Poppins' phone ringing thinking it might have been Meriel's mother, she answered it only to be surprised by a Welsh accent. Meriel listened, like a typical nosey parker, "No, that's no good, we have

a fundraiser tomorrow. We need to get her up to the summit." Poppins slowly looked over towards Meriel as she hung up the phone.

"Was that Mummy?" curious why Poppins looked so sad.

Poppins heart felt so heavy, she tried to put on a brave face and thought quickly how she could tell Meriel the bad news but with a positive twist. "Err, no sweetheart, it was the train station. The steam train that we have booked for tomorrow has broken down, so we have had to cancel our ride."

Meriel interrupted Poppins mid-sentence: "What, we can't go up Snowdon? What was the point?" Poppins felt sick inside and tried to calm Meriel. She pointed out that it hadn't been a waste of time because she had achieved her swim challenge and Mr Kruze and Ross had achieved their cycle challenge, Snowdon was just a small part of the triathlon. "Meriel, at least it broke down tonight and not tomorrow when we were on it, how scary would that be?" said Poppins, but Meriel glanced down at Sam who rested on the table beside her glass.

"What about Sam's new home? We promised to get him onto the mountain Poppins, we promised!"

"You are right, we did promise and that's what we will do, Plan B." said Poppins as she took Meriel's hand to comfort her.

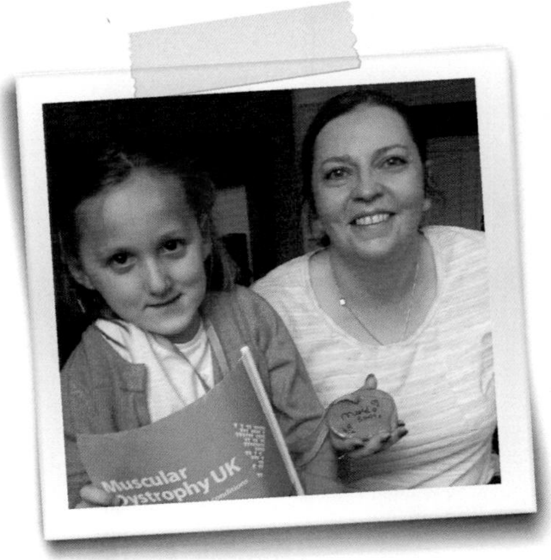

As they discussed Plan B a lady approached them. "I overheard your conversation, I am so sorry to hear that your train has been cancelled. Here's the twenty pounds that you need to take you over the fourteen thousand donated already Meriel, I think you all deserve it."

Fiona's kind words that night really lifted Meriel's spirits and helped her find her positive attitude once again.

"Well, Plan B it is then!" announced Meriel with a hint of positivity;

even though she had started to feel a little overwhelmed by the fact that everything had gone wrong since their arrival.

The rest of the team had soon joined them in the restaurant: "If Poppins can piggyback Sam and me as far as possible, could the Three Musketeers please take Sam up to the summit?" she asked with one of her smiles.

Mr Kruze with his usual positive attitude was definitely up for the challenge even with sore legs. "We won't let you down Meriel."

It was this motivating attitude that had encouraged Meriel. Mr Kruze always smiled as he ran around the school in his runner bean fashion. Even Sam noticed there was something different about him, something that Sam couldn't put his finger on. Mr Kruze was quietly competitive and had a spark that encouraged others to be the best that they could be.

Little did they know at the time, but later that night they discovered that Mr Kruze had had an adventurous life in the golfing world before his life as a teacher.

The team briefly shared their past achievements, including Poppins' surprising life through martial arts.

Sam found it intriguing how Meriel always bonded with such people. "You are very lucky Meriel, you need to carry on being strong and as Poppins and Mr Kruze say, become the best you can be. Keep making yourself proud, that's all that matters." Meriel blushed and snuggled Sam into her neck.

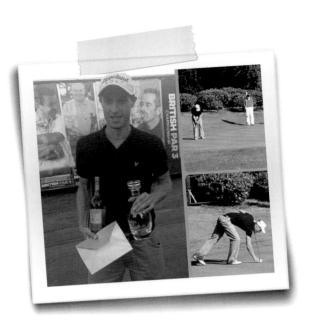

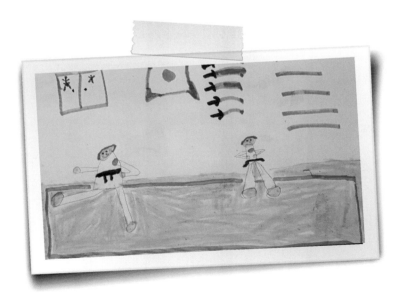

Chapter 7 - The Unlucky Hours

CHAPTER 8
THE LONGEST NIGHT EVER

After they had all shared their own adventurous tales whilst travelling to Wales, Jennie checked the weather at the summit for the next day and the men organised their bicycles.

The boys were disappointed, bicycles were supposed to be kept in the shed provided or they would need to keep them attached to the bicycle rack on the car. "I don't think so," exclaimed Ross, "I am not putting Betsy in the shed, someone might steal her."

Mr Kruze agreed "Yeah, maybe your Bat Bike could fit inside our locked car?"

"And risk someone breaking into my car? Ermmmm no way!" interrupted Jennie.

"I am going to sneak her into my room, no one will notice if I remove her wheels," winked Ross.

Sam agreed: "Let's face it guys, it has been a bit of an unlucky evening so far, it's not worth the risk."

"It has been an evening of bad luck," agreed Poppins, "my bank card doesn't seem to work on the hotel machine either, arghh!" To be safe the men sneaked the bicycles into their hotel rooms.

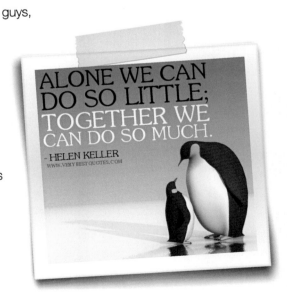

ALONE WE CAN DO SO LITTLE; TOGETHER WE CAN DO SO MUCH.
- HELEN KELLER
WWW.VERYBESTQUOTES.COM

Luckily, the lift was fixed before bedtime which allowed Meriel upstairs in her wheelchair. Poppins gave Meriel a relaxing bath before bed and secretly hoped that it would have calmed her excitement, but with little effect. Meriel was still chatting away until late, reminiscing about all of the funny moments from that evening. Poppins on the other hand was exhausted and ready for an early night. Meriel snuggled her little tiger, he gave her special courage; he fitted in her hand perfectly and she squeezed him if she was ever nervous. Tiger had been with her at the WellChild Awards as well. Sam was all cosy, snuggled down to sleep inside Meriel's hat, beside an organised pile of clothes ready for the next morning's adventures.

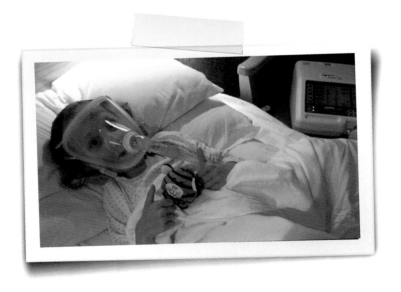

"Goodnight Meriel, goodnight Sam." Poppins sat in the dark for a while until Meriel eventually settled into a sound sleep. Poppins was also restless, it looked like Sam would only get halfway due to time limitations. Poppins texted her good friend Katie and began to plan "Plan C - how to get Sam up to the summit." After all, she had promised.

PLAN C WITH KATIE

Katie had agreed to walk Snowdon with Anna-Marie during the October school holidays several weeks later. They would find where Mr Kruze had hidden Sam at the half way point and continue walking him to the summit and place Sam where he belonged. Katie and her older siblings were the first family that Anna-Marie had cared for (1994). It was Katie's parents that introduced Anna-Marie to Meriel's family, who had local connections in 2012.

The noise of Meriel's ventilator machine that helped her breathe at night, made a horrid continuous sound and then there was the alarm if her face mask moved on her face, all kinds of weird and wonderful sounds were heard. "ARGGHH!" complained Poppins. She plugged in her earphones and placed a cushion over her ears to dull down the noise and eventually drifted off into a light sleep, keeping one ear listening for Meriel.

Ross also struggled to sleep and then the dark clouds eventually burst, DRIP, DRIP, DRIP. He heard the rain in the drainpipe outside his bedroom window all night with its varying pace. Poppins also woke up with the noise of the rain, but she got such a fright, feeling as though she was being suffocated. The pillow that she had used to cover her ears had slid on to her face. "Arghhh!" she yelled, as she quickly threw the pillow to the floor. When she sat up in bed to recover, she glanced over at Meriel who must have had a dream because she had kicked her feet out from under the covers. "Three o'clock, oh dear, it's going to be hard in the morning," yawned Poppins as she plugged in her earphones once again.

Just as Poppins drifted off to sleep, Meriel called for help. "Poppins, can you do bubbles?" She had a very sore tummy with trapped wind.

Poppins had already done the magic bubble trick, which helped remove the wind, several times that night. Not surprisingly it was a long time before Poppins got back to sleep and she was extremely tired when she was woken in the morning by a sweet little voice: "Is it wake up time yet?"

Chapter 8 - The Longest Night Ever

CHAPTER 9
SNOWDON HERE WE COME

Poppins took a long time to wake up, even when her alarm went off, she bashed it onto snooze mode several times. "We better get up," said Meriel, who was so excited and tried to motivate Poppins.

"Yes, you are right, we have lots to do before we meet Jennie and the men downstairs," agreed Poppins as she threw her first leg reluctantly out of the bed.

Poppins had her breakfast on the run whilst she got Meriel ready. Her phone rang unexpectedly: "Morning, it's Mr Kruze, can you two be ready in thirty minutes?"

"Oh, what's wrong?"

Mr Kruze carried on to explain how he and Jennie had got up early and had gone straight to the train station in the pouring rain, to see on the off chance if someone had cancelled their ticket on the other train due to the wet weather. Luckily there were two spare seats and Mr Kruze quickly bought them for Meriel and Poppins. "There won't be room for Walter, her wheelchair though, will she manage?" Poppins couldn't believe the miracle after the unlucky night that they had had. With lightning speed, she encouraged and helped Meriel to get ready more quickly.

MERIEL'S EATING HURDLE

Meriel doesn't eat much, to maximise her food intake, she had an operation to fit a special belly button (gastrostomy - peg tube). A small feeding tube is attached to it, allowing her to have most of her nutrition in the form of a homemade smoothie administered directly into her tummy. Sadly, phlegm and wind continue to upset her tummy, leaving her feeling sick and uncomfortable every morning and often wakes several times during the night.

"But what about the team?" Meriel was in a dilemma, she had to choose between going up to the summit without the rest of the team or to stay with them and walk as far as they could.

"Meriel, I am sure Mr Kruze would think you were very brave if you carried me up the mountain," explained Sam, hoping that she would choose to take him to the very top.

Before long they were making their way to the station, Meriel securely strapped onto Poppins' back and Sam around Meriel's neck. Mr Kruze led the way carrying cushions for the train.

Jennie quickly caught up with them, having failed to raise Ross from his bed.

Luckily, she made it in time to wave Meriel off at the train station. "Toot, toot!" went the old diesel engine as it pulled the carriage up the first steep hill.

Sam was frightened, but he soon relaxed when he noticed that as the lake got smaller and smaller in the distance, the train got closer to the top.

In the meantime, Ross had managed to get himself organised and quickly ran down to the station to catch up with the others. They all looked forward to their walk up the Llanberis path. It wasn't long before the trio had overtaken several families with children that moaned: "Are we there yet?"

By the time the team had approached a gate which marked the official start of the path, they were out of puff. Jennie suggested that they stretch their calves, which were knotted like rugby balls from their cycling.

"Aw that feels better." Mr Kruze's legs had suffered a little.

"See, you should have stretched out in the lake," smiled Jennie.

The team reminisced how well everyone had done when they trundled on. "Every stage has been awesome," commented Mr Kruze, "Hard work, but awesome. From the organising, doing our challenges, to the tremendous amount fundraised."

They agreed and were all very pleased that Meriel had managed to get her train ride up the mountain which allowed her to complete the final

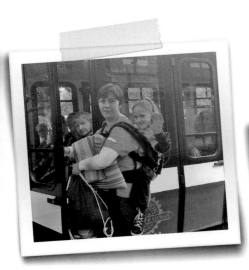

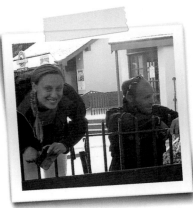

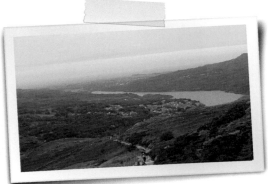

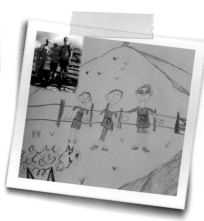

part of their Dream Stone Triathlon. Happy, yet a little sad that the team challenge was nearly over.

Meriel, Poppins and Sam were so excited when the train chugged up the mountain. The surrounding hills became more rugged and the road below through the valley looked just like a pencil line. Sam was amazed when he saw the sheep that munched so close to the track. Suddenly Poppins yelled: "Look, I can't believe it, a Highland cow" She loved Highland cows and was surprised to see one halfway up a Welsh mountain.

The other passengers were very interested to hear about Sam's journey and were so impressed with the team's bravery. Their travel companions were a lovely couple called Bob and Jane. "Do you mind if I ask why are you wearing fancy orange t-shirts?" asked Jane. Meriel explained about the Dream Stone Triathlon. Bob and Jane listened attentively to Sam and Meriel's adventures and were very impressed and couldn't believe that Sam had travelled all the way from Cornwall to achieve his dream. "Everyone has been so brave" commented Jane.

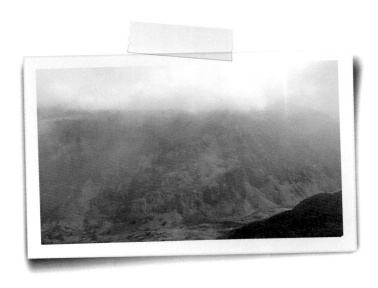

"I am impressed that no one has given up" chipped in Bob, "I would have stayed in bed for a long lie-in if my train had been cancelled."

"Bob, the difference is that Team MAP-N are not lazy like you," joked Jane, everyone laughed.

The train had stopped abruptly. Meriel and Sam held their breath, worried in case the train had broken down. Poppins wondering what was happening and looked outside. The fog had started to get thicker but she was still able to see that they had stopped on a section of double track.

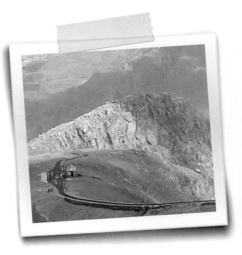

"Oh, it's okay, we have stopped at the passing area, Clogwyn station. There must be another train coming down so we need to wait here to allow it to pass." All the passengers waved out of the window when the trains smooched past each other.

The last climb had been the steepest, everyone had slid out of their seats. Poppins used her arm like a seat belt for Meriel. "Arghhh, help Poppins," chuckled Meriel nervously. Poppins tried her best to keep Meriel and Sam secure, even though she also struggled to stay in her seat. It was only when Poppins looked out of the window that she realised the train track was pinned so close to the cliff edge which explained their very steep climb. Meriel and Sam were worried in case the train slipped off the track and tumbled down the mountain.

Trying to distract Meriel from her fearful thoughts, Poppins said cheerfully, "Hey do you realise that we are climbing Snowdon in the year of it's one hundred and twentieth anniversary, how cool is that!?"

"Really?" smiled Meriel. "That's amazing!"

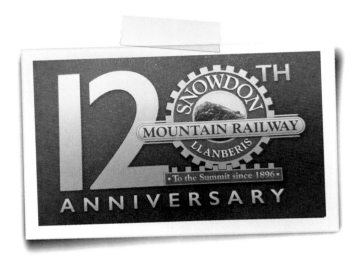

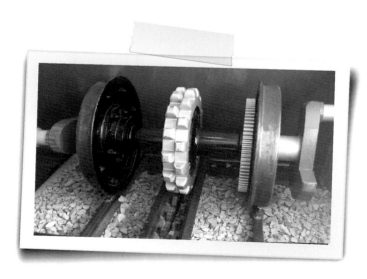

CHAPTER 10
SUMMIT'S UP

As the train pulled up towards Hafod Eryri, the summit visitor centre and café, through the dense fog and mist they saw more walkers who struggled to walk up the last section of steep rubble and shingled path alongside the train track. Poppins decided at that moment to return one day and actually walk Snowdon, it had also been on her Dream List. "As much as I have enjoyed travelling with you guys, I feel the walk needs to be done to achieve a tick on my Dream List."

"Yes, you can come and visit me," said Sam with a huge loving grin.

"Deal," agreed Poppins.

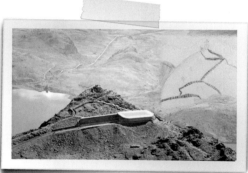

"We are here!" shouted Meriel excitedly, then reality struck her and she whispered, "I am really scared, it's so foggy, what if we fall off the top?"

"Let's just take our time and see how far up we get," with her warm smile, Poppins said the magic words: "Let's do this!"

Jane had kindly helped Meriel back into the sling and she was once again comfortable on Poppins' back. Even though Sam hadn't seen a thing because of the fog he was still quietly excited. They had very little time left to get to the summit, find Sam a perfect spot on the mountain and say their goodbyes before the train left to go back down.

"Hurry!" ordered Meriel, worried about being left up at the summit. "We only have thirty minutes."

Poppins saw the ladder of steep steps that led to the summit in front of her. And was glad that they had practised piggyback not using the hand rail on the stairs at home. Poppins found her dragon spirit and, aware of the time, charged ahead. They passed several walkers who must have thought she was a mad woman to have carried a child on her back to the top.

Sam slowly realised that as exciting as the adventure had been, he was going to have to say goodbye to his best friends. No one had given him so much love and done so much for him in his life. Tears dripped onto his cheek. He had had such an emotional day.

Meriel held Sam close as the steps appeared to finish and the ground level off.

"Oh, look Bob, the little girl is looking for a home for her Dream Stone, let's help her," suggested Jane. Together they began to search for the perfect spot for Sam's new home, they even hung him on a rock like a Christmas decoration, but Meriel thought the wind might blow him away. Eventually she saw the perfect sheltered spot with a little patch of bright green grass that had grown in between the stark grey rock.

"Here, what do you think Sam?" He would be sheltered from the cold, icy wind and hidden from the walkers, but on a clear day he would have an amazing view.

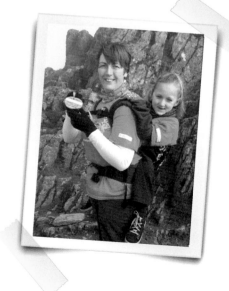

"I love it Meriel thank you." Sam and Meriel then had a quiet moment together, he snuggled into her neck and told her to be brave and to keep moving forward with her own dreams. "Remember, NEVER GIVE UP! Be proud of yourself." Meriel felt emotional, "Bye Sam, I love you," Meriel reluctantly gave Sam to Poppins who removed the orange ribbon that he had been wearing throughout the triathlon.

Poppins gave him a kiss before she placed him gently in his new home.

"I am going to miss you 'Wee Man'" said Poppins in her Scottish accent. "You may be wee, but you will leave a huge hole in my heart. You have helped Meriel so much, we will never forget you."

As Meriel and Poppins started to walk back down the steps Sam called them back "Meriel stop! You must go up to the Trig Point." Sam had noticed that Meriel hadn't actually reached the end, behind him he had seen more steep steps that lead up to the Trig Point, 'Snowdon's crown'.

Poppins, Bob and Jane all turned around. "Oh look, only a few more steps, you may never get the chance again Meriel," encouraged Bob.

"Bye Team MAP Nemaline, proud of you both" shouted Sam with a lump in his throat as he watched the girls walk towards the steps.

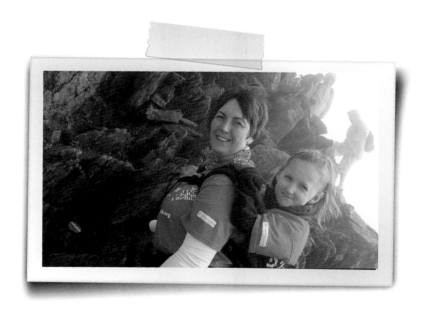

They both waved, but couldn't bring themselves to say goodbye so they smiled and blew him a kiss instead. Poppins confidently stepped forwards to face the last climb, only to be met with a sudden drop off the cliff edge on her right. The wind had got stronger and the fog thicker, how she wished for a handrail. It was a bit scary but she tried not to show her fear to Meriel. "Come on Poppins!" said Meriel who loved the easiness of her part in the summit adventure. "We don't want to miss the train. Let's do this," she giggled as she found it funny that she had used Poppins' Magic words.

"Don't worry Poppins, I will be right behind you, only another few minutes climb," encouraged Bob. Jane had gone in front. Poppins walked up three narrow steps that continued to spiral towards the summit. She had tried to avoid the cliff edge, which meant she hugged the inside of the curved corner of the steps. The steps were narrower and uneven underfoot. Meriel's position on Poppins' back pulled her to one side, it made Poppins feel very unbalanced. A weird sensation had come over her, a sickness deep within and her legs suddenly felt weaker and resembled jelly.

"Oh, I ccaaann't," stuttered Poppins. Her fear of heights had overwhelmed her at this awful moment, however, she knew inside her heart that she had to continue. The team had come too far for her to give up now. Poppins, not happy with the situation, decided to use her hands and feet, walking like a bear the rest of the way up.

"Come on Poppins, you are doing great, you are fine," called Jane from above.

Meriel struggled to breathe because of the new walking style. "I can't breathe" she groaned on the last few steps from the top.

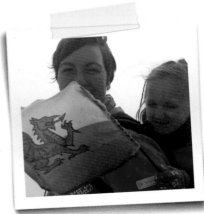

When Poppins heard Meriel's cry for help, she crawled a bit faster and grasped onto Jane's arm at the top. She still felt a bit giddy and balanced herself holding the Trig. "We did it Meriel, we are at the top of Snowdon."

"Yes," stammered Meriel as she recovered from the crawl.

Meriel looked around but was unable to see much because of the thick fog, except for the steep drop to the steps below. "Well, we managed to climb up Meriel, but how on earth are we going to get down?" Poppins' legs continued to tremble a little from the height and narrow standing space.

Poppins suggested that Meriel came out of the sling, she thought it would be safer if they bum-shuffled down the steps.

"NO," screamed Meriel, now scared herself.

"Well Meriel it's not worth the risk, if I fall, you get hurt. Do you understand?" snapped Poppins rather anxious about the time ticking past as she started to undo some clips of the sling, Bob stopped her with a better idea.

"If I went first you could hold onto my bag."

"Yes, and your other hand could hold my walking stick," suggested Jane.

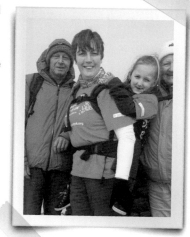

Poppins carefully watched her footing as they slowly went down the steep narrow part together. She was worried about spraining her ankle, how would they have driven back home? Thankfully it was a one-way system and the steps going down were not as scary.

Poppins and Meriel were so relieved to be safely back at the café and thanked

Bob and Jane as they hugged them goodbye. Bob and Jane had decided to walk back down the mountain rather than travel back by train.

There was just time before the train for the girls to quick march to the shop, they decided to buy a keyring each as a memento.

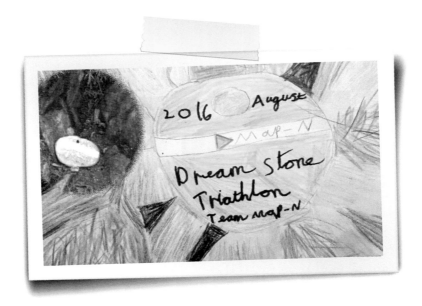

CHAPTER 11
WHAT GOES UP, MUST COME DOWN

Poppins and Meriel looked at each other in disbelief when they heard a seagull squawk as it flew above them. Both girls smiled thoughtfully hoping that it was Sam's friend Gavin, reunited with him on the mountain.

The toot of the train shattered their thoughts.

"Going back always feels quicker Meriel," said Poppins who tried to make conversation but Meriel was looking out of the train window at the views of the mountain tops and hidden lakes, in a world of her own.

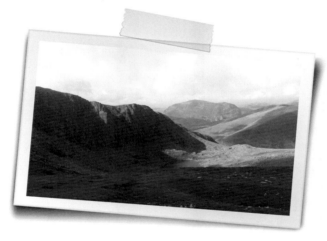

"Let's keep our eyes peeled for our team t-shirts, we may see Mr Kruze and the others." All of a sudden Meriel's ears pricked up like a rabbit.

"Oh yeah, I will look out this side of the train, if you look out of the other side please?" She looked a lot happier when she thought about her teammates.

The steep slope wasn't as scary on the way back down as they knew what to expect. Meriel felt reassured that they were not going to jump off the track, now that she knew that the cogs were doing a good job and helped keep everyone safe.

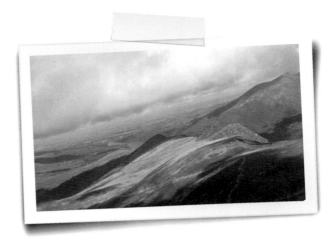

Whilst Meriel and Poppins were on their final part of the Dream Stone Triathlon, Mr Kruze, Jennie and Ross had had their legs put to the test on the footpath. It never stopped climbing, with some very steep parts. There was a favoured corner at the top of a hard climb, a popular rest point with walkers. Here they rested on the large boulders and admired the view of the distant lake.

Just as Jennie jumped back down from her boulder she was almost run over, not by a car but a fell runner!

"That runner must be crazy, they must have started very early to have made it to the summit and be running back down already!" Jennie was surprised.

Ross agreed "Yes, there are some really keen people Jennie, perhaps we should try that next year?" winking at Mr Kruze.

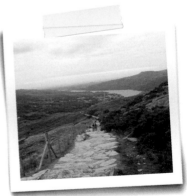

"Or how about trying that Ross?" Mr Kruze pointed to three men who carried their mountain bikes on their shoulders, sweating and out of puff. "Bet you can't wait for the journey downhill on your bikes guys?" Mr Kruze asked enviously. Without the energy to speak they just nodded and smiled. Jennie shook her head "I hope you are only joking? What crazy ideas you have."

Half way up Snowdon there was another resting place, a shelter. The long walk around the side of the hill wasn't so bad, but in fact you had to be careful where you stepped because the path was made of big boulders.

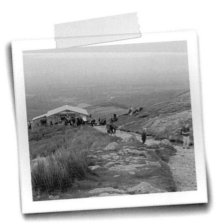 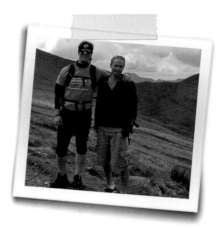

"Take those hands out of your pockets!" snapped Jennie as she flicked Mr Kruze's shoulder, "You should know that walking with your hands in your pocket is dangerous, especially when walking up a mountain." Mr Kruze quickly withdrew his hands, embarrassed because he did know, but it had become a bad habit of his.

Ross chuckled as he walked away. "As Arnold Schwarzenegger said: 'You can't climb the ladder of success with your hands in your pockets'."

As it had been so busy at the shelter, they found another large boulder to rest on and ate some of Jennie's tasty energy bars. "I hope Meriel is okay?" said Jennie as she looked at her watch.

"She would have been to the summit by now and probably on her way down. Keep an eye out for the train," suggested Ross.

On the train, Meriel and Poppins had been orange t-shirt spotting. They had noticed several walkers wearing orange t-shirts, but not their team. As they approached the half way point, they had noticed a cluster of orange when Poppins suddenly recognised Mr Kruze who was madly waving to attract their attention. Poppins lifted Meriel up so she could see them. Poppins shouted over the noise of the train to the other passengers, "Can you all please wave to the rest of our team, we have raised £14,000 for charity."

The passengers all waved as the train slowly chugged by. Meriel was so excited that she wanted to share the summit news with them. "Can we get off the train for five minutes to speak to Mr Kruze?"

"I don't think we can Meriel, sorry." But the train driver had heard all the commotion in the carriage and slowly applied the brakes and stopped.

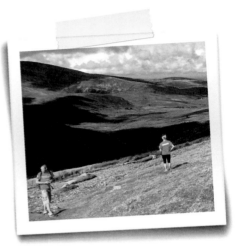

"I can't stop long, there is another train behind me, be quick." Poppins climbed out the carriage and ran towards the others carrying Meriel and their belongings rather haphazardly.

"We did it!" shouted Meriel as loud as she could. Meriel started to tell them the whole story from the beginning, when suddenly there was a toot and they turned to see the train moving.

"I am sorry" shouted the train driver. Meriel stopped mid-sentence when she saw the train move downhill into the cloud of fog that had started to emerge.

"Stop!" she cried. Poppins comforted her and told her that they were all together now and she would still be safe with everyone taking turns to carry her down the mountain.

"Can we just phone Prince William, he flies rescue helicopters, doesn't he?" pleaded Meriel.

Mr Kruze trying not to laugh at her sweet suggestion, encouraged her to enjoy the adventure. "You're mountaineering Meriel, I doubt your friends have done that and certainly not as part of the most amazing team ever, Team MAP Nemaline." Meriel gave him a little smile and they made their way down the mountain.

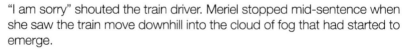

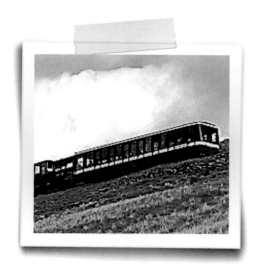

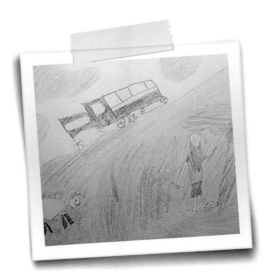

CHAPTER 12
DREAM STONE TRIATHLON ACCOMPLISHED

Poppins was puzzled by what she saw emerging from the fog on the path ahead of them. "What's that? The Highland cow again?"

"I don't believe it," whispered Mr Kruze, as they all stared at the creature blocking their path. "I think it's Pumpkin." Through the fog the little Shetland pony climbed the path towards them and neighed with excitement that he had found Mr Kruze at last.

"How could he have followed us?" said Ross in disbelief. Pumpkin hadn't liked being left after their football game and had barged his way through the hedge. He had followed their scent like a dog, all the way to Snowdon.

"You are unbelievable Pumpkin," said Mr Kruze as he ruffled his mane. Pumpkin approached Meriel and Poppins. Mr Kruze felt a little nervous because Pumpkin was sometimes naughty and nibbled, but Pumpkin was so gentle and had rubbed his nose up and down Meriel's leg and then edged his bottom in front of Poppins, repeating this several times.

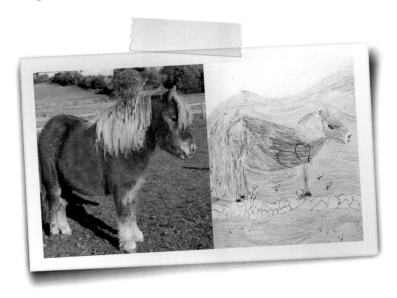

"I think he is trying to tell you that he wants to carry Meriel." suggested Jennie.

Meriel looked a little nervous, but excited at the thought. "Can I?"

Jennie held Pumpkin's head in case he bolted when Meriel sat on him, while Mr Kruze and Ross were nearby to help if needed. Poppins gently and slowly placed Meriel on his wide back. He turned his head and licked Poppins' hand reassuringly as if to say: "I will keep her safe." Jennie tied her scarf around his neck and slowly led him down the path.

When they returned to the hotel Mr Kruze arranged to keep Pumpkin in the paddock next to the hotel garden until his sister could come to take him home. He had rung his sister to reassure her that Pumpkin was safe and had been the hero when he led them all safely back into the village. Meriel and Poppins kept Pumpkin company, while the others prepared to go home.

Pumpkin loved Meriel, he sniffed and nuzzled her. "Stop Pumpkin, that's tickly," she giggled. Meriel promised that she would visit him once they were all back home. "Goodbye my hero, be a good boy."

Poppins gave him a rub on his forehead and also thanked him for leading them all safely down the mountain.

The two men took a long time to get their precious bicycles strapped safely onto the car. Ross had brought lots of bubble wrap which he bandaged around Betsy the Bat Bike's frame. It kept her

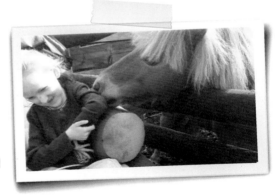

safe from scratches and clunks. Oh dear, thought Poppins. This must be a serious bicycle crush "Come on guys, Meriel is waiting for you all in the garden."

The team were rather subdued as they talked in the garden before going their separate ways. They had mixed emotions, feelings of anti-climax

and tiredness, yet excited with all that they had accomplished.
The team were also overwhelmed when donations continued throughout
the following month.

https://uk.virginmoneygiving.com/MAP-Nemaline

Poppins had a gift for all her teammates, the most perfect triathlon
medal of achievement that had been kindly arranged with the help of
another of Meriel's supporters, 'Trophy-man John'.

TROPHY MAN JOHN

Poppins takes Meriel to see 'Trophy-man John' at his Trophy Centre
in Witney, when she attains her swimming goals. He engraved
anddonated Meriel's first trophy, John loves the fact that she
continues to achieve her goals and his whole family now continue
to encourage her.

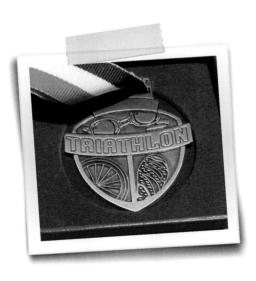

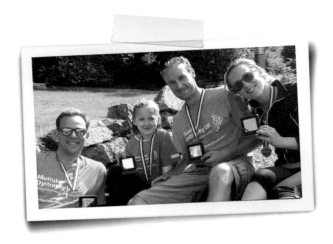

As they celebrated and reminisced in the sunshine, Jennie noticed that Meriel looked a little glum. She was lost in thought thinking about Sam, how he had travelled all the way from Cornwall to reach his dream home and had made it with the help of his friends. Jennie thought a song might cheer Meriel up.

"We started with a great tune, so I think it's only right that we finish with it." Meriel and Poppins' hearts fluttered on hearing the first few bars of their favourite WellChild tune 'Hold my Hand'.

"Perfect Jennie, just perfect!" agreed Poppins. Music had played such a large part of Meriel's journey.

THE ADVENTURE HOWEVER, DOESN'T END HERE FOR MERIEL AND TEAM MAP NEMALINE. THERE WILL ALWAYS BE A DREAM TO CATCH AND A DREAM LIST TO TICK.

EPILOGUE
IF THEY CAN DO IT, SO CAN I!

Meriel's Inspirational Heroes

In 2012 Meriel watched the London Olympics and Paralympics, it was a huge eye opener to see what others can do and what can be achieved. Meriel began to have famous inspirational heroes. In her school work, she mentioned that she wanted to "Dive like Tom Daley and swim like Michael Phelps." Meriel was also smitten by Alexis Sanchez, the Arsenal footballer. At the WellChild awards, both Alexis and Theo Walcott were part of a surprise video message for Meriel.

"I love you Meriel, a kiss for you."

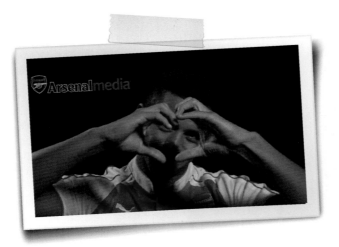

Mr Kruze had organised for GB Rower and Olympic Gold medallist Alex Gregory to come to school to speak with the children. To his surprise 'Meet an Olympian and hold an Olympic medal' was on Meriel's Dream List. Meriel was able to talk privately and have her photograph taken with Mr Gregory, holding his very heavy medal, a definite highlight. They discussed various points, including the importance of healthy food for everyone, especially Olympians. He reminded her to never give up on her dreams. Mr Gregory explained that he started his sporting career as a swimmer before reluctantly trying rowing, and admitted that he had also had several unsuccessful experiences. "That's what makes you stronger, because you learn from it." Talking to Mr Gregory gave Meriel a huge boost. She thoroughly enjoyed shouting encouragement at the television when he achieved his second Olympic Gold at the 2016 Olympics in Rio, over and above being five times World Champion.

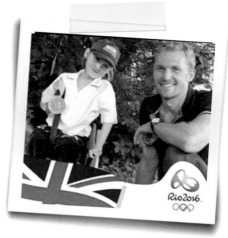

It is difficult to find a healthy life balance and juggle time between jobs, education, training, competing, coaching, not to mention family and trying to maintain a social life or relationship. It becomes even harder when there are enormous health issues causing uncertainty in the future. Meriel has been lucky to know two incredible woman that do just that. They have inspired her and made her realise that life from a wheelchair is not only paper, pen and puzzles, but sport is accessible as well.

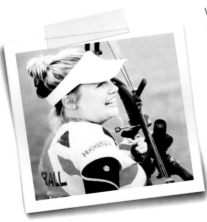

Chloe Ball-Hopkins was also diagnosed with Nemaline Myopathy, like Meriel, but has complications with a bone condition called Arthrogryposis. This means she had no hips and her feet didn't grow in the correct direction. After many operations, this was corrected and eventually she managed to get up onto her feet. Chloe, with her fierce determination, didn't let any of this hold her back. Like most people who have been struck with health issues, they fight back with plenty of spirit.

Chloe's salvation was sport and she had many experiences and successes through a variety of activities. She however, found a passion for archery for which she represented Great Britain in 2014. Chloe has broken and set world records during her career, European bronze being one of her finer moments.

Chloe is currently an ambassador for Muscular Dystrophy UK, the charity that supports a wide variety of muscle disorders and the families who live with them.

Meriel met Elizabeth Grinnell (Liz), at a school talk about wheelchair basketball. She had been born a premature twin with heart valve problems (Pulmonary Stenosis) and developed Spastic Cerebral Palsy Diaplegia as a result of a traumatic birth. In her late teens, Liz's doctors then discovered a hole in her heart, but this didn't stop her. Liz tried a variety of adaptive sports. She excelled at javelin and shotput, with several National gold medals and records to her name.

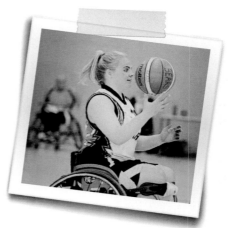

Just prior to Liz's first major competition achievement in 2012 (UK School Games) she suffered three consecutive heart attacks and was put into a medically induced coma. As a result, she unfortunately had to forfeit her place at the London 2012 Paralympic Games. She had thirteen hours of work on her heart, then six weeks on life support. This operation not only saved her life, but gave her the confidence to keep dreaming and the appreciation that we only have one life and to grab those dreams with both hands and do your upmost to make them come true. Liz took first place that memorable day in London at the UK School Games.

Liz is now an ambitious wheelchair basketball player with the Warwickshire Bears, promoting the fact that anything is possible.

These two determined young women who continue to fight health complications are currently training hard, working towards Tokyo 2020 Paralympics, focused on competing for their place on the GB team once again.

Epilogue

Chloe and Liz have both used their experiences to support charity work and encourage others to believe that life does go on and giving up doesn't need to be an option. They have been presented with awards for their dedication for their supportive roles within their community and inspiration to those whose hearts they have touched.

With more than a decade between our Paralympian hopefuls and Meriel, they still have a lot in common. Having a zest for life, great humour, even though their health issues have been acute at times, they never give up. Seeking perfection in everything that they do, making their dreams come true whether that is on the sports field or life in general, paving the way forward for the next generation.

When Team MAP Nemaline shared their previous experiences with each other, Mr Kruze revealed how he had been a talented youngster at golf and progressed to have a professional competitive golf career for several years before he trained to become a teacher. Having achieved several significant wins, sacrificing normal life to follow his dreams.

The team knew that Anna-Marie had been a child carer for many years, but were shocked to learn that alongside her heart-warming role, she also had been successful at Karate. Anna-Marie had trained for over twenty years as a Shotokan karate instructor and international competitor, attaining her 'Yon Dan' (4th Black belt) in Japan in 2004.

Meriel loves listening to Anna-Marie's karate stories and diaries. She especially enjoys looking at the photos and Anna-Marie's international medals. Anna-Marie had learnt a lot about life through her karate career and used many of those lessons to motivate Meriel, 'never giving up,' being lesson number one.

Enormous gratitude goes to all those that have inspired Meriel and continue to do so, teammates and beyond.

Meriel's life has been enriched by having contact with such inspirational people.

Support and a positive spirit is extremely important for anyone going through difficult times, however with uncertain paths due to health issues, support and inspiration can make the journey slightly lighter for everyone. Like leading them through a dark tunnel by the hand whilst pointing the torch, it helps them to see the possibility of stepping forward together.

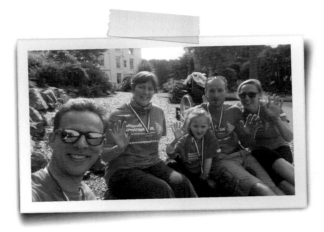

Team MAP Nemaline thought that they were only helping Meriel put a tick on her Dream List, but the reality is the whole experience has had a very significant positive impact on Meriel's life, which has been overwhelming to witness.

'DON'T BE AFRAID TO DREAM BIG AND FOLLOW YOUR DREAMS WHEREVER THEY MAY LEAD YOU. OPEN YOUR EYES TO THEIR BEAUTY; OPEN YOUR MIND TO THEIR MAGIC; OPEN YOUR HEART TO THEIR POSSIBILITIES.'
- JULIE ANNE FORD

If Meriel and her team can do it, so can you. Free your imagination and most importantly enjoy your journey forward with family and friends.

DARE TO DREAM

Let nothing hold you back from exploring your wildest fantasies, wishes and aspirations.
Don't be afraid to dream big and follow your dreams wherever they may lead you.
Open your eyes to their beauty; open your mind to their magic; open your heart to their possibilities.

Dare to dream,
whether they are in colour or in black and white,
whether they are big or small, easily attainable or almost impossible,
look to your dreams and make them become reality.
Wishes and hopes are nothing until you take the first step towards making them something!

Dare to dream,
because only by dreaming will you ever discover who you are,
what you want and what you can do.
Don't be afraid to take risks, to come involved, to make commitment.
Do whatever it takes to make your dreams come true.

Always believe in miracles
and always believe in you!

BY JULIE ANNE FORD

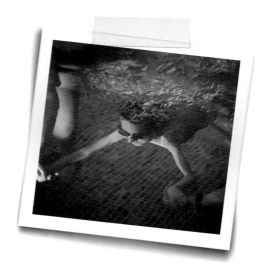

MERIEL'S DREAM LIST ACHIEVEMENTS 2017...

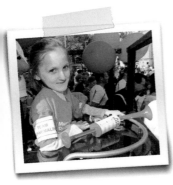

OXFORD T&G 10K
RACE STARTER

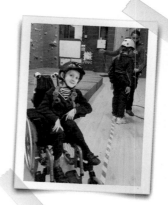

CLIMBING WITH FRIENDS

LOVED SKIING

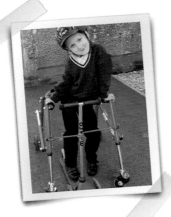

'ZOOTERBOARDING'

PARALLEL LONDON
INCLUSIVE 5K

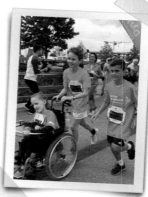

LINKS

BUY MORE COPIES FROM:
thedreamstonespirit.org

MAP NEMALINE:
musculardystrophyuk.org/get-involved/
family-funds/funds/map-nemaline

WELLCHILD:
WELLCHILD.ORG.UK

MERIEL'S AWARD:
https://goo.gl/HoVwBh

SPEAR CHARITY - PUMPKIN:
spearcharity.org.uk/page12.htm

SNOWDON MOUNTAIN RAILWAY:
snowdonrailway.co.uk/pages/
journey-to-the-summit

OXFORD SLING LIBRARY:
oxfordslinglibrary.co.uk

WITNEY TROPHY CENTRE:
witneytrophycentre.com

WALKOPEDIA:
https://goo.gl/ZJf7gi

ALEX GREGORY:
alexgregorygb.com

CHLOE BALL-HOPKINS:
chloeball-hopkins.weebly.com

ABSORB EDUCATION:
absorbeducation.co.uk

KITEBROOK PREPARATORY SCHOOL:
kitebrookhouse.com

**WARWICKSHIRE BEARS
WHEELCHAIR BASKETBALL :**
bearswbc.co.uk/players-wwbc

DISABILITY SNOWSPORT UK:
disabilitysnowsport.org.uk

BORDERS SHOTOKAN:
bordersshotokan.com

BARONS EDEN GROUP:
baronsedengroup.com

WYATTS GARDEN CENTRE:
wyattsgardencentre.co.uk/about-us

SCHOOL NOTICES:
schoolnotices.co.uk

AXICON LABELS:
axiconlabels.com

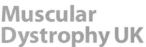

MAP Nemaline
www.musculardystrophyuk.org/map-nemaline

SOCIAL MEDIA

CONTINUE TO FOLLOW, LIKE AND SHARE
OUR STORY AND ALL OF OUR NEW
CHALLENGES ON SOCIAL MEDIA.

TDSSPIRIT1

THEDREAMSTONESPIRIT.ORG

Lightning Source UK Ltd.
Milton Keynes UK
UKRC01n0114100518
322372UK00001B/2

* 9 7 8 1 9 9 9 9 5 4 3 0 7 *